I0423025

Healing Salve:
15 Lessons How to Make a Herbal Salve + 15 Best Recipes

Table of Contents

* * * * * * * * * * * * * * * * * * * *

Introduction Must Have Salve!

Even in today's highly compartmentalized society, there are still some things that we can not always buy right off the shelf of the grocery store and pharmacy. So let us take a moment to step away from the ready made, one size fits all solutions of modernity, and turn again to the natural world, to reclaim the healing remedy that it can provide. Because as extensive research has shown, every single ailment that the human body may suffer—is at its root—caused by some sort of lack or deficiency.

By using herbal salves we are simply replenishing our bodies of what they really need. If you have a bad sunburn for example, this means that you have lost a lot of important nutrients that have been burned out of your skin, the best way for you to heal from this condition then, is to replenish those burned out nutrients by applying a salve such as Aloe Vera directly to the affected surface. Using herbal salves is not a complex science, but it is stunningly exact in its measurements and propensity to heal.

Herbal salves help us to tweak and adjust the constitution of our own bodies at will, allowing us to treat all aches, pains, and irritations by stimulating our own body chemistry through contact with natural medicinal herbs. The use of herbal salves is a medicine that lay physicians of been prescribing for centuries. Even today, many modern therapeutic practices are putting a lot of stock in natural, herbal salves, in their medical practice. Rather than ingesting more pharmaceuticals that mainly mask the deficiencies that make us sick, learn to apply the 15 herbal salves in this book in order to meet any need that your body may have.

Chapter 1: Learn to Rub Some Salve in Your Wounds

Have you ever heard the saying, don't rub salt in your wounds? While this is meant for advice, to not dwell on painful situations, when it comes to herbal salves, you can indeed alleviate many painful situations by learning to do just that. By rubbing specialized healing salves into your cuts, scrapes and burns you can greatly expedite the healing process, while soothing any discomfort you may feel.

Herbal Ashwagandha Salve

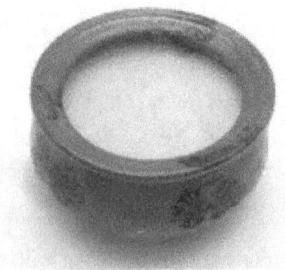

Ashwagandha has an astounding propensity to heal. Known as an "adaptogen" this herbal salve when applied to open wounds helps to enhance the body's own natural healing process, kick starting the formation of platelets, and allowing wounds to bind back together. To create your own Herbal Ashwagandha Salve simply mash this herb into a dusty paste, and keep it stored in a sealed container until you need it. In order to apply this salve, just rub the paste over the wound either with your bare hands, or with a clean q-tip or other sterile instrument.

I can remember a time that I was on vacation out hiking with my wife when I tripped and fell in a ditch. (Great way t start a vacation right?) As I sat up I then realized that my clumsy bumbling not only earned me embarrassment but also severely scraped my knee, as I could see blood spurting out of my ripped jeans. My wife then remembered the Herbal Ashwagandha Salve she had stashed in her backpack and handed it to me. And that stuff was like magic.

As soon as I applied it—to a gaping wound no less—the bleeding stopped, and much of the stabbing pain subsided to just a dull ache. I wasn't the most comfortable, my pride was hurt, but I was able to limp back to camp without incident. Eve more than that, thanks to my Herbal Ashwagandha Salve I knew that I wouldn't have to stay up at night worrying about infection. Herbal Ashwagandha Salve is always great to have on hand. So be prepared for any situation, and stock up on this healing salve.

Healing Grapefruit Salve

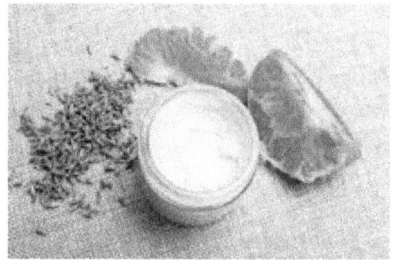

If you fall off your bike and skin your knees, or otherwise find yourself afflicted with cuts and abrasions, your go to source of healing should be a ready made batch of Grapefruit Salve. In order to make your own Grapefruit Salve, drip about 18 drops of Grapefruit oil into a medium sized saucepan set on high heat. Now add 8 drops of beeswax and allow these two ingredients to meld together. You can usually tell just by looking at the concoction how well it is melding together. If it looks clumpy and is overly bubbling, this is a clear indication that it needs to be stirred together better.

But if the blend seems to have a streamlined, uniform surface free of lumps, then you can rest assured that your Healing Grapefruit Salve is well on its way to becoming a powerful and potent blend. Seeing this, continue to stir the contents of the pan thoroughly for another 15 minutes, now turn your burner off and allow the pan to cool. Once sufficiently cooled, pour the mixture into a sealable container and store in a safe place. The next time you get scraped and cut during the course of your day just apply this salve directly to the skin. You will see the difference almost immediately. Just a little bit of this Healing Grapefruit Salve goes quite a long way.

Herbal Dandelion Salve

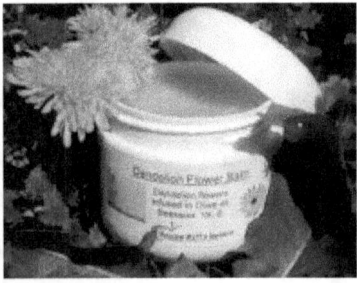

Dandelions can be found just about anywhere, they grow in most people's backyards. But I bet you never imagined that you could use these simple little weeds as a home-grown treatment for open wounds and sores. As it turns out, Dandelions contain a natural chemical agent that upon contact with wounds instantly serves to stimulate the formation of platelets in the bloodstream, allowing scabs to more easily form, greatly speeding up the patient's recovery time. I learned this first hand when I was a small child playing in my grandmother's yard.

My grandparents lived out in the country far from many of the more traditional trappings of society. One day I stepped on a piece of broken glass, and after a quick round of screaming and crying, my grandmother came out to see what the commotion was. Do you know what the first thing this old lady did to help her grandson? Grab a band aid? Use hydrogen peroxide?

Nope! None of those! She simply reached down and pulled up a dandelion right out of the ground and started working its petals into my cut foot. The bleeding seemed to stop almost instantaneously. So believe me, never doubt the power of Herbal Dandelion Salve! Just like your grandmother used to tell you, pick your dandies and save them for another day!

Antiseptic Garlic Salve

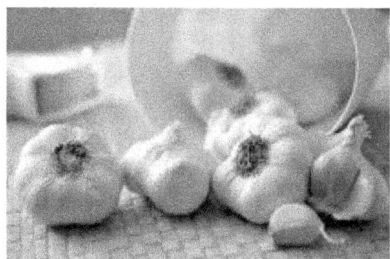

If you are ever far away from home and severely injure yourself, the number one concern that you should have is disinfecting the wound, because even minor wounds if left untreated can become terribly infected. In order to avoid this you need to apply a good antiseptic. And as it turns out, one of the best antiseptics that nature could ever supply is that of everyday garlic. Most of us are more used to using garlic to season our food not our wounds, but it's true, just a small application of garlic at the wound site can clean out the area and stave off infection.

Garlic has many immune boosting and antiseptic properties and this herb is so effective it only takes a small amount for it to work. Garlic has been used for this purpose for thousands of years; many times it was used quite successfully as field dressing for wounded soldiers. Known to prevent gangrene, garlic has saved the life of many troops on countless battlefields all over the planet. The best way to apply this garlic is to smash it into a dusty paste and then simply rub it right into the skin. This Antiseptic Garlic Salve will then get to work, clean out your wounds, and work to keep you safe.

Herbal Lavender Salve

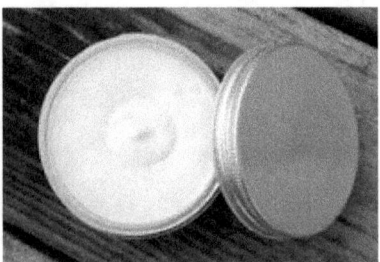

My wife loves lavender; she tells me that just the fragrance of this herb makes her feel good. And many others would concur with this assessment; there is just something intrinsically soothing about lavender. When applied directly to the skin, it can also do much to soothe any irritation that erupts on the dermal layer. If you find yourself break out with a bad case of rash for example, just apply some herbal lavender salve to the troublesome area and it will be able to counteract and treat the surface contaminants until they disappear completely from your skin.

Herbal Lavender Salve also works well to moisturize and clear up skin blemishes such as acne. I've known several people that have used this healing herb for just such a purpose. But whatever the irritation, or even painful wound, Herbal Lavender can fix it for you. In order to make your own Herbal Lavender Salve, take some essential lavender oil and mix it with a vegetable oil base. Thoroughly mix, or shake these ingredients together and then apply a small amount to the area that troubles you. As this healing salve works its magic you will soon be feeling a whole lot better! Herbal Lavender Salve soothes while it heals your wounds!

The Very Vera Healing Salve

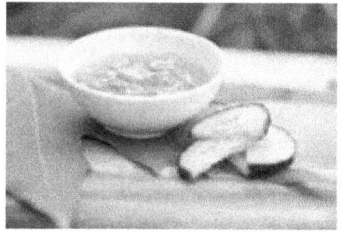

Aloe Vera is a true wonder herb, and when applied as a healing salve it can do wonders for you and any burns or wounds that you may have been afflicted with. While Aloe Vera Gel is common, and can be store bought, it is a simple matter to create your own. You can either grow your own Aloe Vera Plant, or purchase a fresh Aloe Vera leaf from your local health food store. But however you obtain your very own leaf of the Aloe Vera Plant, the next step is to take a knife and cut that leaf open.

Once the leaf has been sufficiently peeled, take a spoon and simply scoop up the gelatinous material on the inside of the leaf. Collect as much of this precious aloe as you can and then put it in a separate container. You then have the option of applying this aloe direct, or slightly diluting it with a good base oil. Either way, this potent salve will still be highly effective. I prefer to dilute mine just to make it last longer. But either way, whenever you get burned, or otherwise wounded, just apply this healing salve and you will be in great shape.

It is the for the treatment of sun burns that you are probably most familiar with this herb, and yes it does have quite a soothing affect on burns. When applied to a burned area of skin you can feel the coolness of the Aloe Vera as it absorbs toxins from your skin, and alleviates much of your pain and suffering.

The chemicals in Aloe Vera work like a sponge taking out of your body what it doesn't need while simultaneously moisturizing the burn and introducing healing agents. Having that said, if you plan on going to the beach any time soon, be sure to pack a hefty does of the Very Vera Healing Salve with you!

Chapter 2: Healing Herbal Salve for those Painful Aches!

We are a culture beset with constant aches and pains, there are chiropractors on every corner and regardless of our occupation many of us wake up feeling as if we had spent the night being slammed by NFL linebackers! As minor as some of this may seem at first, it is these chronic aches and pains that can lead to major disabilities in life.

If you are suffering from chronic pain like this, there is no reason to suffer any longer. And there is also no reason to be addicted to prescription medication just to get through the day. With healing herbal salves you can save yourself a lot of money, pain, and suffering. This chapter will show you how you can use healing herbal salve to get rid of those painful aches once and for all!

Healing Turmeric Powdered Salve

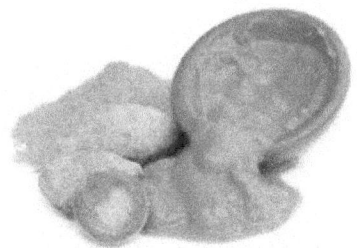

If you do very much cooking, you are probably more familiar with turmeric as a staple ingredient in dinner recipes rather than an integral part of a healing salve. But if you suffer from the aches and pains of chronic arthritis, a small dash of turmeric could do you a whole lot of good. Turmeric has long been known to be able to work its way right into the inflamed joints that tend to suffer so much from arthritis.

Turmeric has a little known ingredient named "curcurmin" that immediately fights inflammation upon contact. For hundreds of years, local medicine men, and backyard pharmacists have actively prescribed and recommended the use of Turmeric for just such problems. Whatever your aches and pains may be, Tumeric is specially suited to take care of them.

If your ankles hurt, rub it into your ankles, if your back hurts, rub it into your back. All of these ancient holy men kept a bit of turmeric around just in case. And just as Turmeric worked so well for so many people suffering in the past, it can still work for your own aches and pains just as well today!

Herbal Valerian Salve

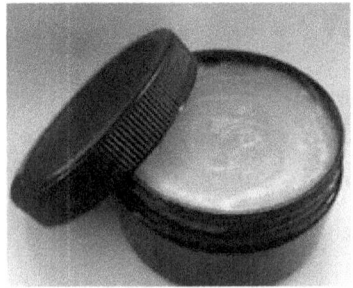

The root of the herbal Valerian plant can be used to treat many aches and pains of the body. Herbal Valerian Salve is especially well suited in the treatment of cramping and other spasmodic problems of the arms and legs. Just grind a fresh batch of Valerian root down into a fine dust and then rub it into the skin. Strategically place this healing salve wherever you are feeling these uncomfortable pains. You should soon feel a slight tingling sensation as a result of the contact.

Herbal Valerian Salve works by sending an instant signal to your nervous system, telling it to relax cramps and spasmodic muscles. If you don't plan on growing this herb yourself, most wellness shops are well stocked with Valerian root. Just buy yourself a batch of it, blend it down in your blender and apply the resulting paste to your aching and spasmodic pains. This Herbal Valerian Salve will make those cramps and muscle spasms a thing of the past.

Ginger Based Herbal Healing Salve

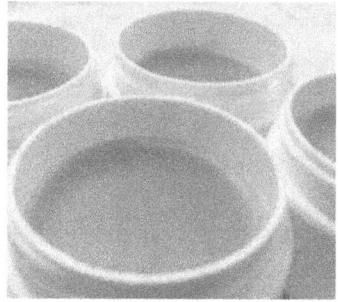

Ginger, yet another common ingredient in cuisine, is also plays an important role as a healing salve. Ginger is a powerful healing agent when it comes for every day aches and pains. Carrying natural anti-inflammatory properties, Ginger can almost instantaneously reduce the effects of inflammation wherever it is applied. So if you have these kind of issues, you should definitely give it a try.

And preparing this salve couldn't be simpler, quicker than you can build a gingerbread house, you can have yourself some Ginger Based Healing Salve. In order to prepare this recipe, just take some fresh ginger, throw it in your blender, put it on high and thoroughly blend this healing salve into a fine paste. Now just find a good place to store this healing salve and use it as needed.

Herbal Devil's Claw Salve

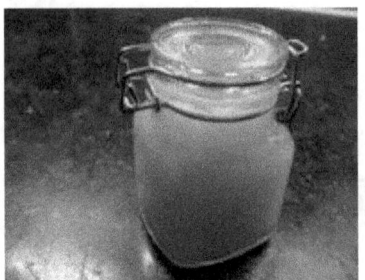

Although it has a rather hellish moniker, Herbal Devil's Claw Salve can do wonders when it comes to a bad backache! This salve stops the pain right at the source! And even better than that, the nourishment that the skin absorbs from this herb serves to replenish many of the body's diminished resources that cause many backaches in the first place! Herbal Devil's Claw Salve works to give you back the balance that your body needs in order to be healthy and pain free.

Many people don't realize this, and often enough physicians won't tell you, but the majority of our aches and pains that we face can be all traced back to some kind of nutrient deficiency in the body. Well, with Herbal Devil's Claw Salve, you can finally a treatment that actually gets to the root of the problem rather than simply masking the symptoms! In order to use this salve, simply it down to a fine paste and apply directly to the skin. I take this stuff wherever I go!

Healing Salve of Herbal Burdock Root

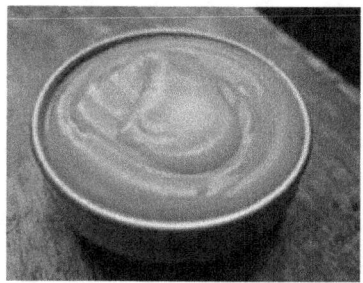

Burdock root is a powerful herb and it has been known to have a wide variety of benefits. But chief among these benefits is this herb's amazing knack for alleviating stiff and uncomfortable joints. There is nothing worse than waking up, or in my case going to sleep, with stiff, uncomfortable joints. I've had this problem for a while now and I find that simply applying this salve on the elbows and knees before I go to bed, allows me to wake up rejuvenated in the morning. Goodbye stiff and aching joints! Burdock has the cure!

In order t make your own batch of Healing Salve of Herbal Burdock Root, simply obtain some fresh, herbal burdock root. If you plan on foraging for this plant, just know that it is most prevalent in spring and it tends to be somewhat pinkish and purplish in appearance. Otherwise you can buy this herb from any health food store, already prepared and ready for your use.

Once you obtain this herb simply grind it down into a dusty powder and apply it directly to your stiff joints. The active agents in this healing salve will then immediately get to work in relieving your aches, pains, and stiffness. This powder also makes for great foot baths, just dump it in warm water, relax, and let the Healing Salve of Herbal Burdock Root do all of the rest!

Chapter 3: Herbal Salve and Your Immune System

The human immune system is the most impressive firewall you could ever imagine. Blocking viruses and other threats in such real time speed that even MacAfee would be jealous! Having that said; the immune system is a complex apparatus, comprised of multiple agents, working together in order to safeguard you from harmful outside pathogens. Since are immune system requires this teamwork in order to run efficiently, we can quickly become severely compromised if even just one aspect of our built in defenders begins to malfunction.

At times it can become hard to keep all the moving parts of our immune system running in sync, it is when this happens, when our immune defense system becomes unbalanced that we end up with the flu, colds, and even worse maladies. But once again, since invariably, a poor immune system response is due to a lack of specific nutrients in the body, these failures can be counteracted and safeguarded against with the right application of herbal medicine. This chapter provides you with some of the best ways to utilize herbal salves in order to maintain immune health.

Immune Healing Rose Salve

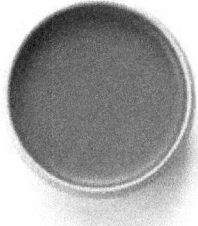

Just the smell of the rose flower can induce elevated mood, and enhance immune health. This is no accident, because this herb happens to be full of very special chemicals that promote overall well being and health. In order to create your own Immune Healing Rose Salve, simply gather up a typical rose flower and then grind it down into a fine powder.

You can then mix this herb with a carrier oil and store it in an airtight container. Now whenever you feel your immune system begin to take a dive, you can simply apply this healing salve. This is especially important during the cold and flu season, just as you would normally take a flu shot; consider taking an herbal dose of this Immune Healing Rose Salve. Your immune system will thank you for it!

Herbal Chamomile Salve

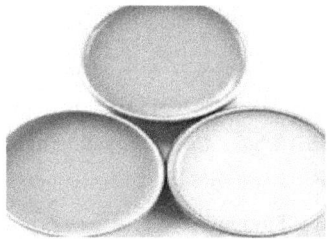

Chamomile has many relaxing properties, but it is also provides a good boost to immune health. Chamomile has an amazing ability to reach all the way down to the circulatory system, helping to regulate blood flow and pressure. This is a great way to reboot a sluggish immune system. In order to apply this herbal salve, simply mash it into a fine paste and paint it right onto the skin. After applying this healing salve I often feel a warm flush and feel good in the knowledge that my blood is getting refreshed, and redirected in a minor that will support my overall immune system health. Herbal Chamomile Salve is always worth a try.

Healing Cat's Claw Salve

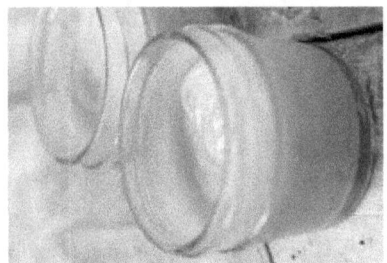

Cat's claw is a true classic in the field of herbal therapy and for good reason. This herb is able t boost the immune system like no other! Cat's Claw has been in use for centuries in order to utilize its amazing ability to increase the body's white blood-cell count. Cat's Claw also strengthens the immune systems reaction time, allowing for faster disposal of outside threats and pathogens. This healing salve provides a direct barrier against disease and infection.

This herbal salve has even been tremendously helpful in HIV patients, bringing some back from the very brink, by increasing white blood-cells when other treatments have failed. If you need any extra help at all to get your immune system in good running order, I would suggest trying this Healing Cat's Claw Salve. Simply mash this herb down into a paste and rub it right into the skin. After doing this you, whatever it is that you are going through, you will find yourself on the mend; and your immune system will be on the rebound very soon.

Herbal Echinacea Healing Salve

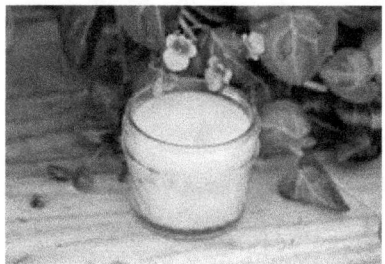

Echinacea has a wonderful way of promoting immune health. Echinacea naturally fights of most bacteria and viruses immediately upon contact. If you are feeling even the slightest bit under the weather, just apply some Echinacea directly to the skin, and the absorbed nutrients will work to directly boost your immune health. Just smash this herb down into a paste and you can use it as much as needed. I've even made the sweet smelling Echinacea into a kind of hand lotion before, a great compliment to my antibacterial hand soap during the flu season!

I tend to use Herbal Echinacea particularly in the colder winter months. I find that it is a great way to boost my immune system when I really need it. As testament to how powerful this stuff is, my father used to make Echinacea based poultices and would where them around his neck when he came down with the flu or colds. It was a goofy sight to see the man walking around the house with a herbal necklace on, but sure enough he would be healed of all that ailed him the next day. And a good Herbal Echinacea Healing Salve can do the same for you!

Chapter 4: Some Direct Methods for Creating a Salve Base

Now that we have discussed at length the main 15 types of herbal salves you can use, in this chapter let's go over some of the more direct methods in which you can create a base in which to deliver your healing salve. Follow these instructions well, and you will be able to create a wide variety of salve bases for your very own herbal, healing salve treatment.

Using Herbal Infused Oils

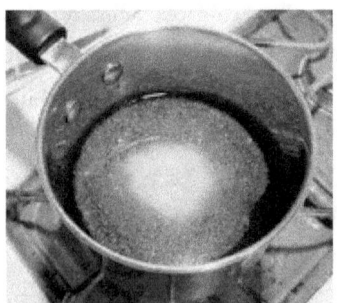

In order to create an herbal infused oil base in which to carry your salve the first thing that you need to do is fill a medium sized jar about 1/3 of the way full, next pour out the oil that you are using and with this addition you should be able to fill up your jar completely. Now simply cover the jar with an air tight lid and store it in a temperate location (around 80 degrees) for a few weeks.

At the end of a few weeks your herbal infused oil should be well marinated, taking on a strong and potent aroma. This concoction is ready to be used as a working salve base. I have find that herbal infused base oils work best with roots, such as Burdock Root. But how you apply this salve base is completely up to you. It is precisely this very versatility of use that makes herbal infused oils, such a great platform.

The Double Boiler Method

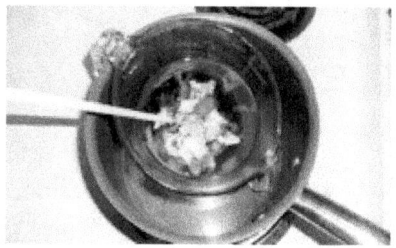

In this method we start out by chopping up whatever herbs we are using into small pieces. Now take these pieces and put them in a double boiler. Next, pour your oil of choice over the chopped herbs and set your boiler on a low heat setting. Now allow this mixture to cook in the boiler for about 35 minutes. During this process it is important not to step away from the boiler, always be vigilant and watch in case the oil gets too hot.

You will have to babysit this brew for at least an hour and a half in order to make sure that it is thoroughly blended and cooked together. Once you have done this, turn off your burner and allow the mixture to cool off. After you have done this you can then strain your oil out by means of a cheesecloth strainer. With the excess oil separated from the herbs place the herbs in a dry cloth and put them off to the side. These herbs can then be used again for later projects so don't lose them. Finally take the oil you have strained and put it in a safe container. This will work as a good salve base for many more herbal concoctions.

Traditional Herbal Salve

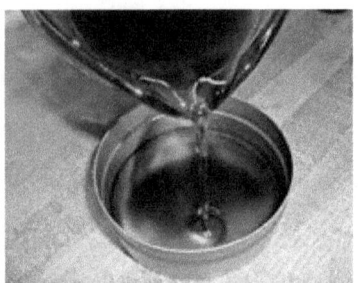

To get started with this one, take 1 cup of an oil base and put it in a glass container. Now place the container in the center of a big pan filled with H2O. Now add about one ounce of paraffin or beeswax and set your burner on low heat. While this is cooking place a spoon in your freezer. I know this sounds strange, but it is actually very important.

You see, the frozen spoon is necessary for use in periodically stirring and checking the structural integrity of the salve. This spoon always you to blend the oil without breaking its bonding potential. Stir the mixture like this periodically for a couple of hours, and then turn your burner off and allow the mix to cool. Once cool, you have yourself a great batch of traditional salve to use as the base for your healing herbs.

Conclusion: There is a Salve that can Solve It!

I used a bit of humor in the heading above, but in all seriousness, I have yet to find an ailment that there isn't some herbal treatment or salve that can't be used to treat it. That's why it is so important for us to get back to nature, and the natural treatments that it can provide for us. The human body evolved to live on this planet, whether we realize it or not we are a part of this environment. That means that we are intrinsically linked to the plants and animals of this Earth.

This is why I can confidently say that for any ailment that we may have, there is a cure for it, somewhere in the natural world. All of the nutrients we need, we share and have in common with the flora and fauna of this earth. So the sooner you take the natural route, and begin to opt for herbal based treatments such as healing salves, the sooner you can reclaim control over your biological health. If I have said it once, I will say it a billion times, no matter what problems you may be facing, somewhere out there, there is a salve that can solve it! Thank you for reading!

FREE Bonus Reminder

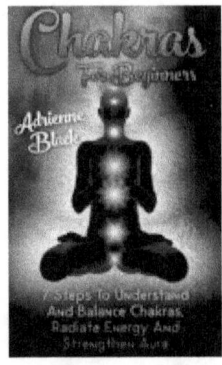

If you have not grabbed it yet, please go ahead and download your special bonus E book *"Chakras for Beginners. 7 Steps To Understand And Balance Chakras, Radiate Energy, And Strengthen Aura"*.

Simply Click the Button Below

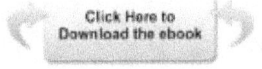

OR Go to This Page

http://lifehacksworld.com/free

BONUS #2: More Free & Discounted Books & Products

Do you want to receive more Free/Discounted Books or Products?

We have a mailing list where we send out our new Books or Products when they go free or with a discount on Amazon. Click on the link below to sign up for Free & Discount Book & Product Promotions.

=> Sign Up for Free & Discount Book & Product Promotions <=

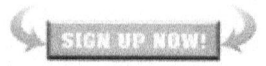

OR Go to this URL

http://zbit.ly/1WBb1Ek